Dr. Demetre Daskalakis's statement on Bird Flu outbreak:

Everything you need to know about the recent outbreak

Harold Muller

All rights reserved. No part of this publication may be reproduced, distributed, or transmitted in any form or by any means, including photocopying, recording, or other electronic or mechanical methods, without the prior written permission of the publisher, except in the case of brief quotations embodied in critical reviews and certain other noncommercial uses permitted by copyright law.

Copyright © 2024 by Harold Muller

Table of Content

Table of Content..3
Introduction...6
   The Importance of Expert Insight in Global Health Crises..9
   Introduction to Dr. Demetre Daskalakis.................. 13

Chapter One: The Emergence of the H5N1 Bird Flu17
   Overview of the 2024 Bird Flu Outbreak.................17
   Historical Context: Previous H5N1 Incidents and Lessons Learned.. 20
   The Current Strain: What Makes H5N1 Different?. 23

Chapter Two: Dr. Demetre Daskalakis and the CDC's Role..26
   Who Is Dr. Demetre Daskalakis?...........................26
   His Leadership at the CDC................................... 28
   The National Center for Immunization and Respiratory Diseases (NCIRD) and Its Mission......31

Chapter Three: Dr. Daskalakis's Statement on the Bird Flu.. 36
   Breaking Down Dr. Daskalakis's Official Statement36
   The Key Messages on Risk and Response............39
   The Global and Local Health Implications of H5N1 41
   Addressing Public Concerns and Misconceptions..43

Chapter Four: The Mechanisms of H5N1: How the Virus Spreads... 46
   Understanding Avian Influenza..............................46
   The Transmission Pathways of H5N1.................... 48
   How Infected Animals and Humans Interact...........52

The Role of Backyard Flocks and Animal Agriculture. 53

Chapter Five: Public Health Measures: The CDC's Strategy 56

The Role of the CDC in Managing Outbreaks 56

Surveillance and Early Detection Systems 58

Quarantine, Testing, and Isolation Measures 60

Public Health Guidelines for Communities at Risk. 63

Chapter Six: Regional Impacts: The Case of Louisiana and California 65

A Closer Look at the Louisiana Bird Flu Case 65

Dr. Daskalakis's Role in the Investigation 67

The California State of Emergency: Government Response 69

The Role of State Health Authorities in Managing the Outbreak 72

Chapter Seven: What We Know and What We Don't: The Unanswered Questions 75

Understanding the "Spillover" Phenomenon 75

Why Some Are More at Risk Than Others 77

Research Gaps and the Need for Further Study 80

Dr. Daskalakis's Call for Continued Monitoring and Vigilance 82

Chapter Eight: Risk to the Public: Analyzing Dr. Daskalakis's Risk Assessment 84

How the CDC Determines Risk Levels 84

The Role of Age, Health Conditions, and Exposure... 87

The Reality of Person-to-Person Transmission 91

Chapter Nine: Preparing for the Future: Lessons

from the H5N1 Outbreak... 94
    Global Health Security and Pandemic Preparedness. 94

    The CDC's Long-Term Vision for Handling Avian Influenza.. 96

    Lessons Learned from the 2024 Outbreak and Future Risks... 99

    How Communities Can Prepare for Future Outbreaks... 101

Chapter Ten: Beyond the Bird Flu: Dr. Daskalakis's Broader Impact on Public Health............................ 103

    Dr. Daskalakis's Contributions to Infectious Disease Control.. 103

    Advancing Public Health Policy............................ 106

    The Role of Leadership in Managing Health Crises... 108

Conclusion.. 113

    The Role of Expert Voices in Shaping Public Health Responses.. 115

    Final Thoughts on the Global Health Landscape.. 118

Introduction

In the face of emerging infectious diseases, expert insight has never been more crucial. Global health crises, such as pandemics, epidemics, and viral outbreaks, often present complex and rapidly evolving challenges. The world needs clear, actionable information to understand and mitigate these threats. This is where the expertise of public health professionals, virologists, epidemiologists, and other specialists comes into play. Their roles are indispensable in managing health crises, providing the public with accurate information, guiding government policies, and ensuring coordinated responses.

Historically, many of the world's most significant health challenges, such as the HIV/AIDS epidemic, the 2003 SARS outbreak, and the 2009 H1N1 influenza pandemic, were met with expert guidance and intervention. The experts who guided the response to these crises not only worked tirelessly to manage the immediate effects of the outbreaks but also contributed to the long-term strategies for preventing future health emergencies.

In the case of the 2024 H5N1 bird flu outbreak, Dr. Demetre Daskalakis, as a prominent figure within the Centers for Disease Control and Prevention (CDC), exemplifies the importance of expert voices in global health. His role is particularly significant as the outbreak poses a potentially dangerous threat to human health. In such situations, the public must rely on the knowledge of experts like Dr. Daskalakis to navigate through the uncertainty, understand the risks, and take the necessary steps to protect themselves and others.

When infectious diseases like H5N1 make headlines, it can be easy for fear and misinformation to spread. Social media platforms, news outlets, and even casual conversations often amplify unverified claims or skewed data. Experts provide much-needed clarity and balance, translating complex scientific information into comprehensible guidance for the public. Their analysis can help dispel myths, calm widespread panic, and foster informed decision-making at all levels, from individual citizens to governmental institutions.

The H5N1 bird flu outbreak has underscored this need for expert insight. While bird flu has been a known threat for many years, new strains like the one currently affecting parts of the U.S. and beyond are raising fresh concerns. These strains, particularly the D1.1 variant, appear to be more contagious and severe than previous versions. The intervention of experts like Dr. Daskalakis is crucial to understanding the nature of these changes and formulating strategies to control them. His statement on the virus, detailing its transmission, risks, and the public health response helps shape the global understanding of the outbreak and informs both individual and institutional actions to reduce the spread of the virus.

The role of experts during a health crisis extends far beyond scientific data. It also includes providing leadership in crisis management, communication, and policy development. As we saw in the case of the COVID-19 pandemic, without clear guidance from public health leaders, communities can become fragmented in their response, leading to ineffective strategies and unnecessary loss of life. Dr. Daskalakis's position at the CDC allows him to offer not just scientific insight but also leadership in terms of public health communication and resource allocation.

In conclusion, the importance of expert insight in global health crises cannot be overstated. Experts provide the necessary scientific and practical knowledge to confront emerging diseases and offer solutions that balance public health, safety, and well-being. Through their leadership, the global community is better equipped to prevent, manage, and ultimately overcome these health threats.

The Importance of Expert Insight in Global Health Crises

Global health crises are increasingly becoming a norm in today's interconnected world. Whether it's the rapid spread of a viral disease like COVID-19 or the emergence of avian influenza strains like H5N1, these crises can have far-reaching consequences on public health, economies, and daily life. During such times, expert insight is crucial not only to understand the complexity of the disease but also to guide governments, organizations, and individuals in making informed decisions. Experts especially those in public health, virology, epidemiology, and other related fields provide a backbone of knowledge that supports decision-making in these challenging times.

At the heart of every global health crisis is the need for accurate, timely, and effective communication of scientific data. In the absence of this expert-led communication, misinformation, confusion, and fear can take over. This is particularly true in a time when social media and instant communication platforms spread news (and rumors) faster than ever before. In moments of uncertainty, when people are most vulnerable, they need trusted voices who can break down the science behind the outbreak and provide clear recommendations on how to protect themselves and others.

One of the key areas where expert insight proves invaluable is in understanding the transmission dynamics of a disease. For example, the H5N1 strain of avian influenza, which has been circulating globally, poses unique challenges for public health systems. The virus is typically transmitted between birds, but it can sometimes jump to humans, resulting in severe illness. The specifics of how and why this happens, which populations are most at risk, and how the virus might mutate are questions that can only be answered through expert knowledge. Dr. Demetre Daskalakis's statement on the ongoing H5N1 outbreak, for example, provides an in-depth understanding of the virus's behavior and its potential impact on human health.

Public health experts also play a crucial role in formulating the response strategies to health crises. This includes coordinating with international health organizations, advising governments on emergency measures, implementing containment protocols, and ensuring the availability of vaccines and medical treatments. During an outbreak, experts help determine the most appropriate interventions, balancing the need for public safety with the realities of resources and potential social and economic disruptions. Dr. Daskalakis's leadership at the CDC during the 2024 bird flu outbreak highlights how experts influence policies aimed at preventing the spread of diseases. His recommendations for protecting vulnerable populations, such as those working with poultry or living in regions with high exposure to wildlife, guide not only public health authorities but also individuals who are at risk.

Moreover, the involvement of experts is vital in the aftermath of a health crisis. Once an outbreak has been controlled, experts analyze the response and make recommendations for improvements. This can include refining surveillance systems, enhancing emergency preparedness, and preparing for future outbreaks. The lessons learned from one crisis help inform strategies to address the next. Public health professionals like Dr. Daskalakis play a key role in ensuring that each crisis becomes a stepping stone to better preparedness in the future.

Finally, expert insight fosters public trust. In times of crisis, people are often frightened and uncertain. Without the voices of respected experts, people may turn to inaccurate or misleading sources for answers. By offering clear, factual, and empathetic guidance, experts help calm fears, reduce panic, and encourage collective action. As the H5N1 bird flu outbreak continues to evolve, Dr. Daskalakis's role in managing public perception through communication remains a critical part of the CDC's strategy.

In conclusion, expert insight is an indispensable asset in managing global health crises. From understanding disease transmission to guiding public health policy, experts are the critical link that connects scientific research to real-world action. Their knowledge, leadership, and communication can mean the difference between a manageable outbreak and a full-scale disaster. As the world continues to face emerging infectious diseases, the value of expert-driven responses will only increase.

Introduction to Dr. Demetre Daskalakis

Dr. Demetre Daskalakis is a leading public health expert with extensive experience in infectious disease control and immunization strategies. As the director of the National Center for Immunization and Respiratory Diseases (NCIRD) at the Centers for Disease Control and Prevention (CDC), Dr. Daskalakis has played a pivotal role in shaping the United States' response to several public health crises. His work has gained widespread recognition, particularly for his leadership during the COVID-19 pandemic and his ongoing efforts to tackle emerging threats like the H5N1 bird flu outbreak.

Dr. Daskalakis's background is rooted in both clinical and public health practice. He earned his medical degree and later specialized in epidemiology and infectious diseases, which paved the way for his current role at the CDC. His expertise spans a wide array of diseases, ranging from influenza and COVID-19 to vaccine-preventable illnesses. In his capacity as director at NCIRD, Dr. Daskalakis is responsible for overseeing the development and implementation of strategies aimed at preventing infectious diseases and promoting vaccination across the United States.

One of Dr. Daskalakis's most notable contributions has been his work in pandemic preparedness and response. During the COVID-19 pandemic, he emerged as a trusted voice, guiding the public and health professionals through an unprecedented global crisis. His clear and data-driven communications helped shape policies on testing, social distancing, and vaccination, all while ensuring that the most vulnerable populations received the attention they needed.

Beyond COVID-19, Dr. Daskalakis's expertise in infectious diseases has positioned him as a key figure in addressing other potential health threats. The ongoing H5N1 bird flu outbreak, for instance, has placed him at the forefront of public health efforts. His statement on the outbreak provided critical insight into the transmission and risks associated with the virus, as well as the CDC's response to the evolving situation. He highlighted the need for vigilance and precautions, especially for those in high-risk sectors such as poultry farming and those in contact with wild birds.

Throughout his career, Dr. Daskalakis has demonstrated an unwavering commitment to public health. His work has not only shaped national health policies but also contributed to global efforts to prevent the spread of infectious diseases. His leadership continues to be instrumental in the CDC's work, ensuring that the U.S.

remains prepared to handle both current and future health crises.

In sum, Dr. Demetre Daskalakis is a highly respected public health expert whose career has been dedicated to advancing our understanding of infectious diseases and improving the nation's preparedness for future health threats. His work is instrumental in shaping both national and international public health responses, particularly in times of crisis, and he remains a crucial figure in the ongoing battle against infectious diseases.

Chapter One: The Emergence of the H5N1 Bird Flu

Overview of the 2024 Bird Flu Outbreak

In 2024, the world has once again found itself on high alert due to the resurgence of H5N1 bird flu. This strain of avian influenza, which was first identified in domestic poultry in 1997, has been circulating in birds for decades, causing widespread concerns about potential human transmission. Although the virus primarily affects birds, particularly waterfowl and poultry, its potential to infect humans has led to significant public health precautions and responses.

The 2024 outbreak of H5N1 bird flu stands out not just because of its scale but also due to the evolving nature of the virus. It is now recognized as having a greater capacity for spillover into humans, potentially causing severe illness or even death. The Centers for Disease Control and Prevention (CDC) and the World Health Organization (WHO) are closely monitoring the situation, focusing particularly on cases where human-to-human transmission is suspected.

This latest outbreak began in regions with significant wild bird populations and commercial poultry farms, particularly in North America and parts of Europe. The primary route of transmission to humans has been through direct contact with infected birds or their excretions. However, with the increasing reports of human cases, experts have grown concerned about the virus evolving in a way that could make it more easily transmissible among humans.

As of late 2024, there have been several reported human cases, the most severe of which occurred in Louisiana, where a person was hospitalized with critical respiratory illness after exposure to infected backyard poultry. This case underscores the growing threat of H5N1 to public health, especially as the virus continues to circulate in wild bird populations and poultry. Dr. Demetre Daskalakis, a leading figure in infectious disease control, has played an integral role in advising the public and health authorities on how to manage this outbreak.

The CDC has issued guidelines for those living or working in areas affected by the outbreak, particularly for those in the poultry industry, wildlife conservationists, and people with backyard flocks. These recommendations emphasize preventing exposure to infected birds, especially as the virus can be spread through contaminated surfaces, air, and water.

In response to the outbreak, governments have implemented various measures to control the spread of the virus, including the culling of infected animals, movement restrictions, and increased surveillance of wildlife. The availability of a vaccine remains uncertain, but efforts to develop an effective vaccine that could prevent human infection are underway.

The global response to the H5N1 outbreak is a reminder of how interconnected the world is in terms of disease transmission. With the constant movement of people, animals, and goods across borders, what begins as an outbreak in one region can quickly become a global health threat. Therefore, the focus is not only on curbing the spread of the virus in affected areas but also on preparing for any potential escalation that might lead to a pandemic.

Historical Context: Previous H5N1 Incidents and Lessons Learned

H5N1 bird flu has a long history of causing global concern. First identified in Hong Kong in 1997, the H5N1 strain of avian influenza was the first known instance of a bird flu virus infecting humans. It caused severe illness and deaths, with 18 reported cases and six fatalities. This early outbreak sparked fears of a pandemic, particularly because of the virus's high mortality rate among humans.

Since 1997, H5N1 has re-emerged in several waves, particularly in Asia, Europe, and the Middle East, where it has been responsible for sporadic human infections. The virus has primarily spread to humans through close contact with infected poultry, particularly in regions where there are large commercial poultry industries and where biosecurity measures are lacking. The virus has also been detected in wild birds, which has complicated containment efforts, as these birds can travel long distances, unknowingly spreading the virus to new areas. One of the most significant outbreaks occurred in 2003, when the virus spread across much of Southeast Asia, affecting millions of birds and leading to the culling of infected flocks. This outbreak also saw a significant number of human cases, prompting the World Health Organization (WHO) to issue warnings about the potential for the virus to mutate and gain the ability to spread more easily among humans. At the time, there were widespread fears that H5N1 could become the cause of a global pandemic, similar to the 1918 Spanish flu, which killed millions worldwide.

In response to the threat of H5N1, governments and health organizations took several steps to limit its spread. International organizations like the WHO and the CDC worked to improve surveillance and reporting of cases, and countries with known outbreaks implemented culling programs, vaccination campaigns for poultry, and travel restrictions. Several vaccines for H5N1 were developed, though they were primarily designed for poultry, not humans.

Despite the heightened fear and extensive efforts, H5N1 did not evolve into a global pandemic. While human infections continued to occur sporadically, the virus did not easily transmit between people, limiting its ability to spread in the population. However, the lessons learned from past outbreaks were invaluable in shaping the response to future health crises, particularly the COVID-19 pandemic.

The H5N1 outbreaks of the past have underscored the importance of early detection, global cooperation, and transparent communication in managing public health threats. Public health experts and organizations learned the value of rapid response mechanisms and the need to develop vaccines and antiviral drugs that could be stockpiled for future use. They also emphasized the necessity of educating the public about how to reduce the risk of infection, especially for those living in or working in close proximity to poultry and other birds.

The 2024 outbreak serves as a reminder that the lessons of past bird flu incidents are still relevant. Although H5N1 has not yet reached pandemic levels, its potential remains a significant concern for global public health. Understanding the mistakes and successes of previous responses is critical in developing more effective strategies for dealing with this and future outbreaks.

The Current Strain: What Makes H5N1 Different?

The H5N1 bird flu virus has evolved significantly since it was first identified in 1997. The 2024 outbreak presents several new challenges that make this strain of the virus different from earlier versions. While H5N1 has historically been primarily a bird-to-human transmission virus, the current strain shows signs of becoming more adaptable and capable of causing more severe illness in humans.

One of the key factors that distinguish the 2024 strain of H5N1 is its increased capacity for human-to-human transmission. Historically, the virus has required close contact with infected poultry to jump to humans. However, there have been reports suggesting that the current strain might be more easily transmitted between humans, which is concerning for experts. While there is no evidence yet of widespread human-to-human transmission, this potential shift has raised alarms.

Another factor that makes the 2024 strain of H5N1 more concerning is its severity in humans. The virus has been associated with severe respiratory illness, including pneumonia, which can be fatal, especially in individuals with underlying health conditions. The Louisiana case, where an individual over 65 with pre-existing medical conditions was hospitalized in critical condition, highlights the increased danger this virus poses. In previous outbreaks, many human cases were milder, but the current strain seems to cause more severe outcomes.

Genetic studies of the virus have shown several mutations in the hemagglutinin (HA) and neuraminidase (NA) proteins, which could allow the virus to better bind to human respiratory cells. These mutations could enable the virus to spread more easily through airborne droplets, as opposed to the more difficult-to-transmit forms that require direct contact with infected birds or their droppings.

The adaptability of the virus has raised concerns among public health experts about the possibility of a future pandemic. While vaccines are being developed, their effectiveness in preventing human infection with the new strain is still under study. Additionally, the virus's ability to mutate means that any vaccine may need to be updated regularly to remain effective against new strains.

The strain's impact on the global poultry industry is another area of concern. Large-scale poultry farming is widespread, especially in developing countries, and H5N1 poses a significant risk to food security. Efforts to cull infected flocks and prevent the spread of the virus can lead to the destruction of millions of birds, further straining agricultural economies already affected by the outbreak.

In conclusion, the 2024 H5N1 strain is different from its predecessors in its potential for human-to-human transmission, its increased severity in humans, and its adaptability. These changes present new challenges for public health organizations and governments, making it crucial to monitor the virus closely and respond swiftly to mitigate the risks of a wider outbreak.

Chapter Two: Dr. Demetre Daskalakis and the CDC's Role

Who Is Dr. Demetre Daskalakis?

Dr. Demetre Daskalakis is a prominent figure in the field of infectious disease control and public health. As the Director of the National Center for Immunization and Respiratory Diseases (NCIRD) at the U.S. Centers for Disease Control and Prevention (CDC), he has played a crucial role in shaping the country's response to various health crises, including the COVID-19 pandemic and the more recent bird flu outbreaks. His expertise, leadership, and commitment to public health have made him an authoritative voice in global health discussions.

Dr. Daskalakis's journey into public health is marked by both a deep passion for epidemiology and a unique blend of experiences. Before joining the CDC, he earned his medical degree and completed extensive training in the field of public health. His early career focused on infectious diseases, with a particular interest in how viruses and other pathogens spread in communities, especially among vulnerable populations. He worked in various capacities that allowed him to explore both the scientific and practical aspects of disease control, including fieldwork in underserved areas.

Daskalakis's reputation in public health grew as he worked on several high-profile projects aimed at controlling infectious diseases. His significant experience includes contributions to the CDC's efforts to combat HIV/AIDS, sexually transmitted infections, and other diseases that disproportionately affect marginalized communities. His expertise extends beyond the technical side of infectious diseases; his ability to communicate complex public health issues to the public and policymakers has made him an effective advocate for health education and preventative measures.

One of his most significant achievements has been his leadership in navigating the challenges posed by emerging infectious diseases, particularly those that have the potential to cause global pandemics. His approach is grounded in science but also focused on community engagement and education. This holistic approach has made him a well-respected public health leader, and his work has earned him recognition both in the United States and internationally.

In the context of the 2024 H5N1 bird flu outbreak, Dr. Daskalakis has been at the forefront of the CDC's response, offering expert guidance and oversight on how to manage the spread of the virus, mitigate its risks, and prepare for potential future threats. His leadership during this crisis reflects his depth of knowledge in infectious disease control and his commitment to protecting public health on a global scale.

His Leadership at the CDC

Dr. Daskalakis's leadership at the CDC is defined by his expertise in managing complex public health emergencies and his ability to coordinate responses to large-scale outbreaks. As the Director of the NCIRD, his role is to oversee efforts related to immunization, respiratory diseases, and other viral infections, including flu outbreaks and bird flu incidents like H5N1. The CDC is the United States' primary agency responsible for protecting public health and safety, and Dr. Daskalakis's leadership has been critical in ensuring that the organization's responses to public health emergencies are timely, coordinated, and effective.

One of Dr. Daskalakis's key strengths is his ability to combine scientific expertise with practical, actionable public health strategies. In the case of the 2024 H5N1 bird flu outbreak, he has been instrumental in developing and disseminating guidelines to mitigate the virus's spread. These guidelines have included recommendations for individuals who may be at risk, such as poultry workers, wildlife conservationists, and individuals with backyard flocks, all of whom are more likely to be exposed to infected birds.

Under Dr. Daskalakis's leadership, the CDC has worked tirelessly to ensure that accurate information is provided to the public. Misinformation, particularly during a health crisis, can lead to confusion and fear, so his efforts to communicate effectively with the media, the public, and other public health organizations have been crucial in managing public perception of the outbreak. He has emphasized the importance of transparency, timely reporting, and consistent messaging to avoid panic and promote effective prevention strategies.

His role also involves coordinating with other agencies and organizations, both domestically and internationally. As the outbreak of H5N1 is a global concern, the CDC's efforts cannot be isolated to the United States alone. Dr. Daskalakis has worked alongside the World Health Organization (WHO), the United Nations, and various national health agencies to track the virus's movement and ensure that containment measures are in place across borders.

Moreover, Dr. Daskalakis has worked on strengthening the CDC's preparedness for future outbreaks. His leadership includes advocating for continued research on vaccines, antiviral treatments, and improved diagnostic tests, all of which play a critical role in preventing the spread of diseases like H5N1. His emphasis on innovation in public health responses has positioned the CDC to better handle future crises, both known and unknown.

In addition to his scientific expertise, Dr. Daskalakis is also known for his ability to manage and inspire teams. The work of the CDC involves numerous public health professionals, including epidemiologists, virologists, and emergency response specialists, all of whom must collaborate effectively to address an outbreak. His leadership style fosters a culture of teamwork, mutual respect, and a shared commitment to public health.

Dr. Daskalakis's ability to provide clear guidance while also remaining open to new information and approaches has been critical in his role at the CDC. As the virus continues to evolve, his leadership has helped ensure that the CDC is responsive to the changing landscape of the outbreak, adapting strategies as needed to protect public health.

The National Center for Immunization and Respiratory Diseases (NCIRD) and Its Mission

The National Center for Immunization and Respiratory Diseases (NCIRD), led by Dr. Daskalakis, is one of the most crucial units within the CDC. The NCIRD plays a pivotal role in preventing and controlling vaccine-preventable diseases, as well as respiratory infections, including influenza, COVID-19, and avian influenza such as H5N1. The center's mission is to ensure that the United States is prepared to handle any infectious disease outbreak, with a specific focus on reducing the impact of these diseases through immunization, surveillance, and public health interventions.

The NCIRD's work spans a wide range of activities, all aimed at promoting public health. It provides expert guidance on immunization schedules, offers recommendations on vaccination practices, and supports research into new vaccines and treatments. The center also coordinates with local, state, and international health agencies to implement strategies for controlling infectious diseases.

One of the key functions of the NCIRD is to manage the U.S. vaccine supply. This includes monitoring vaccine safety, ensuring that vaccines are distributed effectively, and coordinating vaccination campaigns to reduce the incidence of diseases like the flu, measles, and polio. The center also plays an integral role in managing the response to respiratory diseases, such as influenza and COVID-19, by conducting surveillance, collecting data, and analyzing trends to inform public health policy.

The work of the NCIRD has proven especially valuable during health crises. The center's expertise in immunization and disease prevention is crucial in minimizing the spread of respiratory infections, especially in outbreaks like H5N1 bird flu. The NCIRD helps guide decisions on whether vaccination campaigns should be implemented, how vaccines should be distributed, and what additional measures may be necessary to reduce the impact of an outbreak.

In the case of the H5N1 bird flu, the NCIRD's role is critical in providing the CDC with the data and resources necessary to track the virus's spread and recommend preventive actions. This includes making recommendations on which populations should receive the vaccine, monitoring the effectiveness of these interventions, and conducting research to understand how the virus may evolve.

The NCIRD is also involved in the development of new vaccines for emerging infectious diseases. The center works closely with pharmaceutical companies, research institutions, and other government agencies to accelerate the development and approval of vaccines that can prevent diseases like bird flu, which may not have an established vaccine yet. In addition to vaccine development, the NCIRD is involved in advancing diagnostic tools, antiviral treatments, and other public health interventions that can reduce the impact of respiratory infections.

As part of the CDC, the NCIRD has a global reach. In addition to working with domestic partners, the center collaborates with international health agencies to control infectious diseases worldwide. This is particularly important for diseases like H5N1, which can cross borders through the movement of birds, animals, and people. The NCIRD's ability to monitor global trends and share information with other countries allows for a coordinated international response to outbreaks.

In conclusion, Dr. Daskalakis's leadership at the CDC, combined with the mission of the NCIRD, positions the United States to respond effectively to infectious disease outbreaks like the H5N1 bird flu. The center's focus on immunization, disease surveillance, and public health interventions has proven invaluable in protecting public health and mitigating the impact of respiratory diseases. Dr. Daskalakis's role in guiding these efforts continues to be critical as the CDC navigates the challenges of emerging infectious diseases in a globalized world.

Chapter Three: Dr. Daskalakis's Statement on the Bird Flu

Breaking Down Dr. Daskalakis's Official Statement

Dr. Demetre Daskalakis's official statement on the 2024 H5N1 bird flu outbreak offers a detailed overview of the situation, emphasizing the seriousness of the threat while also providing reassurance and guidelines for the public and healthcare professionals alike. As one of the leading voices at the CDC, Dr. Daskalakis's statement was pivotal in framing the response to the outbreak, ensuring that individuals and communities knew how to manage their risks while also minimizing public panic.

At the core of Dr. Daskalakis's statement was the need for vigilance, preparedness, and adherence to established health protocols. He highlighted that, while the current bird flu outbreak in the United States was alarming, it should not yet be cause for widespread fear. The CDC, he emphasized, was actively monitoring the situation, and ongoing research would be crucial in understanding the full scope of the outbreak. His focus was on ensuring that the public recognized the significance of the disease but also knew that risk mitigation strategies were in place.

The statement provided detailed guidance about the nature of H5N1 and how it spreads. Dr. Daskalakis underscored the fact that H5N1 was primarily a disease affecting birds, but its capacity to infect humans had been demonstrated in previous cases, particularly in regions with close contact between humans and poultry. He was clear that human-to-human transmission had not been observed in the current outbreak, although he noted that it remained a possibility that required continuous monitoring.

Dr. Daskalakis also addressed the importance of preventive measures, including limiting exposure to infected birds, proper hygiene practices, and the use of personal protective equipment (PPE) by those most at risk, such as poultry workers and those with backyard flocks. The statement was not only a response to immediate concerns but a call to action for both public health officials and the general public. He stressed the need for continued research into vaccines and antivirals and called for ongoing collaboration with international partners to ensure the global response was unified and effective.

The statement also served as a reassurance to the public, stressing that, while the virus was serious, the risk to the general population remained low. Dr. Daskalakis reminded the public that the CDC, alongside state and local health departments, had protocols in place to respond to outbreaks swiftly and efficiently, and that public health efforts were focused on preventing further spread.

Through his message, Dr. Daskalakis provided a sense of control and clarity in the face of a public health emergency. His statement was balanced, focusing on the facts while offering practical advice and alleviating undue concern. This clarity and leadership were essential in guiding the public's understanding and shaping the health response as the situation continued to evolve.

The Key Messages on Risk and Response

Dr. Daskalakis's statement focused heavily on two key areas: the risk posed by H5N1 and the CDC's response to the outbreak. His message was clear in addressing public concerns, emphasizing the importance of monitoring and mitigating the risk of transmission, particularly among individuals most likely to come into contact with infected birds.

On the risk of H5N1, Dr. Daskalakis made several important points. Firstly, he emphasized that the current strain of the bird flu was not easily transmissible to humans and that there was no evidence of widespread human-to-human transmission at the time of his statement. However, he acknowledged the potential for the virus to mutate and become more transmissible, a point that warranted close surveillance. This created a sense of urgency without fueling panic.

Dr. Daskalakis also underscored the importance of keeping the public informed and ensuring that accurate, timely information was available. He made it clear that while the overall risk to the general population remained low, those who worked with or around poultry especially in commercial and backyard settings needed to take necessary precautions. These included wearing protective gear, avoiding direct contact with sick or dead birds, and ensuring that all poultry were properly handled and cooked.

On the response, Dr. Daskalakis emphasized the robust efforts of the CDC, local public health agencies, and international bodies. He assured the public that the CDC was coordinating closely with state and local health departments, as well as global partners, to track the virus's movement and respond to emerging cases. This response involved extensive monitoring, rapid diagnostic testing, and quarantine measures when necessary.

He also highlighted the CDC's commitment to researching new vaccines and antiviral treatments, as well as preparing contingency plans for the potential spread of the virus. This included the possibility of deploying vaccines and antivirals if the virus were to mutate into a more dangerous form. Dr. Daskalakis reinforced the idea that proactive measures, including vaccination campaigns and surveillance, were key components of the CDC's strategy to prevent further transmission.

By focusing on these two key messages, the risk assessment and the coordinated response, Dr. Daskalakis worked to provide the public with the information they needed to stay safe, while also reinforcing confidence in the health systems in place to manage the situation.

The Global and Local Health Implications of H5N1

The implications of H5N1 bird flu extend far beyond the borders of any single country. While the 2024 outbreak had its epicenter in the United States, the virus is a global threat, and its impact on global health cannot be understated. Dr. Daskalakis acknowledged both the global and local dimensions of the crisis in his statement. On a global scale, H5N1 presents a significant challenge to public health systems. The virus is not confined to any one country or region, and its rapid spread across bird populations can lead to widespread outbreaks in poultry farms and wild birds. This can cause major economic damage, especially in countries that rely heavily on poultry farming as an economic staple. In addition to the economic impact, there is the potential for public health threats in countries with less robust healthcare infrastructure, where outbreaks could spiral into larger-scale epidemics.

Furthermore, H5N1's capacity to mutate and adapt poses an even greater threat to global health. While the current strain is not easily transmissible between humans, history has shown that avian influenza viruses can evolve to facilitate human-to-human transmission. The global health community must remain vigilant, Dr. Daskalakis warned, to prevent a situation where the virus becomes more virulent and harder to control.

Locally, the implications of H5N1 are no less significant. In the U.S., the outbreak has had a particular impact on the agricultural sector, especially in states with large poultry industries. Farmers, poultry workers, and others who are in close proximity to infected birds face heightened risks. Dr. Daskalakis noted that the spread of the virus to commercial farms, in particular, would require swift action to prevent significant loss of life, both human and animal.

The local health implications also extend to public health preparedness. In areas with large poultry populations, local health authorities must be prepared for potential outbreaks, including the use of quarantine measures, testing, and vaccination programs. Dr. Daskalakis stressed that the U.S. CDC's role in supporting state and local authorities through rapid diagnostic testing, protective equipment distribution, and guidance on quarantine protocols would be crucial in minimizing the impact of the virus on local populations.

Ultimately, the outbreak's global and local health implications hinge on cooperation and preparedness. Dr. Daskalakis's statement reflected the interconnectedness of global health security, highlighting that a coordinated response, driven by accurate information and timely action, would be critical in addressing the H5N1 threat at all levels.

Addressing Public Concerns and Misconceptions

A key aspect of Dr. Daskalakis's statement was his emphasis on addressing public concerns and misconceptions surrounding the bird flu outbreak. With any health crisis, misinformation can be as dangerous as the disease itself, and Dr. Daskalakis was proactive in setting the record straight.

One of the most common misconceptions about bird flu is that it poses an immediate and widespread threat to human health. Dr. Daskalakis worked to dispel this fear by clearly stating that, while the virus is serious, the risk to the general population remained low. He clarified that the virus is primarily spread through direct contact with infected birds and their secretions, and the chances of widespread human infection were unlikely under current conditions.

Another common concern was related to food safety. With H5N1 being a disease affecting poultry, many people feared that consuming chicken or eggs could lead to infection. Dr. Daskalakis reassured the public that properly cooked poultry was safe to eat, as the virus is destroyed by heat. He emphasized the importance of following safe food-handling practices, including thorough cooking and proper hygiene, to prevent any potential risk.

Dr. Daskalakis also addressed concerns about the availability of vaccines and treatments. He acknowledged that there was no specific vaccine for H5N1 at the time, but the CDC and other agencies were actively working on vaccine development. He also stressed that antivirals were available to treat the virus and that, with proper medical care, those who contracted H5N1 could recover.

By addressing these and other misconceptions, Dr. Daskalakis helped to keep the public calm and focused on the facts. His communication played a key role in managing public perception and ensuring that people had the correct information to protect themselves and others.

Chapter Four: The Mechanisms of H5N1: How the Virus Spreads

Understanding Avian Influenza

Avian influenza, commonly known as bird flu, is a viral infection that primarily affects birds, although certain strains, such as H5N1, have shown the potential to infect humans and other animals. The H5N1 virus is a subtype of the Influenza A virus, which belongs to the family of Orthomyxoviridae. Influenza viruses are characterized by their ability to mutate quickly, which is why they can sometimes cause large-scale outbreaks and pose significant health threats to both animals and humans.

Avian influenza viruses are divided into two categories based on their pathogenicity in poultry: low pathogenic (LPAI) and highly pathogenic (HPAI). H5N1 is classified as a highly pathogenic virus, meaning it can cause severe disease and death in birds, particularly in chickens and turkeys. HPAI strains are more likely to spill over into humans, as they are more capable of causing systemic infections in various animal species.

The H5N1 virus was first identified in 1997 in Hong Kong, and it gained international attention after it caused an outbreak of human infections in Asia. Since then, the virus has spread across the globe, sparking concerns about the potential for a pandemic. H5N1 can be transmitted among birds through feces, nasal secretions, and saliva, with wild waterfowl often serving as asymptomatic carriers, making it particularly challenging to track and contain.

In birds, the virus is primarily transmitted through direct contact with infected birds or their contaminated excretions. Wild waterfowl, such as ducks and geese, are the natural reservoir for many avian influenza viruses, and they can carry the virus without showing symptoms of illness. Domestic poultry, on the other hand, are more likely to develop severe symptoms or die from the infection, making outbreaks in commercial farms and backyard flocks of particular concern.

While H5N1 is primarily a disease of birds, it has been known to infect humans, particularly those who come into close contact with infected birds. Human infections are rare, but the virus has a high mortality rate among those who do contract it, leading to heightened concern among health experts. In humans, the virus typically causes severe respiratory illness, including pneumonia, and can rapidly progress to organ failure.

Understanding avian influenza is crucial for managing outbreaks and preventing the spread of the virus to humans and other animals. Researchers are constantly studying the behavior of the virus, including its transmission pathways and mutation patterns, to better predict its potential impact and develop effective vaccines and treatments.

The Transmission Pathways of H5N1

The transmission of H5N1 from birds to humans involves several pathways, with the virus primarily spreading through direct contact with infected animals or their excretions. However, the exact mechanisms by which H5N1 spreads to humans are complex, and understanding these pathways is essential for preventing future outbreaks.

1. Direct Contact with Infected Birds: The most common pathway for human infection with H5N1 is direct contact with infected birds. This can occur in poultry farms, live bird markets, or even backyard settings where infected birds are present. The virus is primarily transmitted through respiratory droplets, feces, and saliva. Individuals who handle infected birds or their contaminated products, such as feathers or eggs, are at the highest risk.

Poultry workers, farmers, and veterinarians are particularly vulnerable because they are in frequent contact with sick birds. In some cases, individuals who have had close contact with dead birds, such as those involved in culling efforts during outbreaks, have contracted the virus.

2. Environmental Contamination: In addition to direct contact with birds, H5N1 can spread through contaminated environments. The virus can survive for a prolonged period in the environment, especially in cold, damp conditions. This means that surfaces and materials that come into contact with infected birds, such as cages, feeding equipment, and clothing, can harbor the virus and serve as vehicles for transmission.

For instance, in poultry farms where biosecurity measures are lacking, the virus can spread rapidly through shared surfaces and equipment. Similarly, in live bird markets, where birds from different farms are sold in close proximity, contaminated surfaces and air can contribute to the spread of the virus.

3. Airborne Transmission: While the primary mode of transmission for H5N1 is through direct contact with infected birds, there is some evidence to suggest that the virus can be transmitted through the air. Studies have shown that airborne particles containing the virus can be present in areas where infected birds are housed. This is

of particular concern in confined spaces such as poultry sheds, where the virus can spread rapidly among large numbers of birds.

However, the risk of airborne transmission to humans is less well understood. While there have been some reports of human infections occurring in proximity to infected poultry farms, there is no conclusive evidence that H5N1 can spread easily through the air over long distances or in a manner similar to seasonal flu. Nonetheless, close proximity to infected birds and poor ventilation in certain settings can increase the likelihood of inhaling viral particles.

4. Human-to-Human Transmission: One of the most significant concerns about H5N1 is its potential to mutate and acquire the ability to spread more easily between humans. While human-to-human transmission of H5N1 is extremely rare, it has been documented in a small number of cases, often in healthcare settings where individuals have had close, prolonged contact with an infected person.

In the event that H5N1 evolves into a strain that can be transmitted more efficiently between humans, the potential for a pandemic increases significantly. This is why public health experts are closely monitoring the virus's mutation patterns and preparing for the possibility of human-to-human transmission. In the absence of such mutations, the primary focus remains on preventing animal-to-human transmission through strict biosecurity measures and surveillance.

5. Global Spread via Migratory Birds: Another key factor in the transmission of H5N1 is the role of migratory birds in spreading the virus across regions. Wild birds, particularly those that travel long distances during migration, can carry the virus without showing symptoms. This makes it difficult to track the movement of the virus and predict where outbreaks will occur next. Migratory birds can introduce the virus to new geographic areas, where it may then spread to domestic poultry populations. This is one of the reasons why H5N1 outbreaks have been reported in a wide range of countries, often starting in regions with large populations of migratory waterfowl.

How Infected Animals and Humans Interact

The interaction between infected animals and humans is central to understanding how H5N1 spreads. The virus typically enters the human body through the respiratory tract, but it can also be transmitted through mucous membranes, such as the eyes, nose, and mouth, if a person comes into contact with infected materials.

Once inside the human body, H5N1 targets cells in the respiratory system, including the lungs, where it can cause severe illness. In humans, the infection often leads to pneumonia, acute respiratory distress syndrome (ARDS), and organ failure. The severity of the disease varies depending on the individual's health status and how quickly they receive medical care.

While the risk of human-to-human transmission is low, the interaction between infected animals and humans is still a major factor in the spread of the virus. For instance, when a human becomes infected with H5N1, they may inadvertently spread the virus to others if proper precautions are not taken, such as isolating the infected person and using appropriate personal protective equipment.

The Role of Backyard Flocks and Animal Agriculture

Backyard poultry flocks and commercial animal agriculture play a critical role in the spread of H5N1. In many parts of the world, especially in rural communities, families raise poultry for personal consumption or local sale. These small-scale operations often lack the biosecurity measures seen in large commercial farms, making them more susceptible to outbreaks.

Infected birds in backyard flocks can easily transmit the virus to other animals, including those in nearby farms.

The close proximity of domestic poultry to wild birds further increases the risk of cross-species transmission. As wild birds migrate, they can introduce the virus to areas with large concentrations of domestic poultry, amplifying the spread.

Animal agriculture, on the other hand, involves large-scale poultry farming operations that can house thousands of birds in confined spaces. If biosecurity measures are not strictly followed, the virus can spread rapidly within these farms, leading to significant losses in both bird populations and the agricultural economy.

Farm workers and others involved in poultry farming are at an elevated risk of exposure to H5N1, making it essential for these industries to implement stringent biosecurity protocols, including regular testing, quarantine measures, and the use of protective clothing. Ensuring that both commercial and backyard poultry operations are aware of the risks and take appropriate precautions is key to preventing the spread of H5N1 to humans.

Chapter Five: Public Health Measures: The CDC's Strategy

The Role of the CDC in Managing Outbreaks

The Centers for Disease Control and Prevention (CDC) plays a pivotal role in managing public health outbreaks, especially those caused by infectious diseases like the H5N1 avian influenza virus. As the United States' national public health institute, the CDC is tasked with monitoring, controlling, and preventing the spread of diseases within the U.S. and globally. Its responsibility encompasses surveillance, research, response coordination, and the dissemination of critical health information to the public.

During an outbreak such as the H5N1 bird flu, the CDC's role is multifaceted, encompassing not only direct intervention to contain the virus but also long-term planning to mitigate future threats. This involves collaboration with local, state, and international health organizations, including the World Health Organization (WHO) and the World Organization for Animal Health (OIE). The CDC's efforts are essential in controlling the spread of the virus, minimizing human-to-human transmission, and preventing large-scale public health crises.

The CDC takes an active role in tracking the virus through comprehensive surveillance systems, ensuring timely detection of cases. Additionally, it is involved in issuing guidelines and policy recommendations on how to handle infected animals, conduct screenings at points of entry (airports, borders), and prepare healthcare systems for potential cases of human infection. By providing both technical assistance and leadership, the CDC is a central figure in outbreak response.

Moreover, the CDC coordinates emergency responses, including providing resources such as protective equipment, antivirals, and vaccines when necessary. Their expertise in epidemiology, virology, and infectious diseases allows them to offer guidance on how best to control the disease and reduce its spread in the population.

The role of the CDC extends beyond the immediate response, as it also provides data and insights that inform government actions and shape public health policy. Its work during previous outbreaks, such as the H1N1 flu pandemic in 2009 and the COVID-19 pandemic, has demonstrated the importance of its swift response to emerging health threats.

Surveillance and Early Detection Systems

Surveillance and early detection are the cornerstone of the CDC's strategy in managing outbreaks, including those caused by avian influenza strains like H5N1. Through surveillance, the CDC can monitor disease patterns, identify outbreaks early, and assess the risk to human health. Early detection is crucial, as it allows public health officials to take swift action to control the spread of the virus before it becomes a larger threat.

One of the key surveillance mechanisms used by the CDC is the National Influenza Surveillance System, which tracks flu-like illness across the U.S. This system relies on data from hospitals, physicians, and laboratories to detect spikes in cases of flu and flu-like illnesses. For avian influenza, the CDC also works in close collaboration with state and local health departments, the Department of Agriculture, and international organizations to track outbreaks in both animal populations and humans.

In addition to traditional surveillance methods, the CDC utilizes genomic sequencing to track the virus's mutations. This is especially important with a virus like H5N1, which is capable of rapid mutations. Sequencing allows the CDC to detect potential changes in the virus that could affect its transmissibility or severity, helping predict whether the virus could pose a greater risk to humans.

The CDC also maintains a close watch on outbreaks of avian influenza in other countries, particularly in regions where the virus is endemic or where there is a high risk of human infection. By monitoring global outbreaks and collecting data from international partners, the CDC can assess the likelihood of the virus spreading across borders, making international surveillance efforts critical to preventing global pandemics.

To ensure early detection, the CDC has implemented a variety of reporting and diagnostic systems. These systems rely on both passive and active surveillance. Passive surveillance involves collecting reports from hospitals, laboratories, and health professionals, while active surveillance involves targeted efforts to search for new cases of disease, including visiting poultry farms and other high-risk areas. Early detection helps to implement containment measures such as travel restrictions or animal culling before the virus can spread further.

Quarantine, Testing, and Isolation Measures

Quarantine, testing, and isolation are fundamental public health tools used by the CDC to prevent the spread of infectious diseases, including the H5N1 bird flu. These measures are designed to contain the virus and prevent it from reaching a broader population, particularly in the case of a novel strain that could potentially cause human-to-human transmission.

Quarantine: Quarantine involves the separation and restriction of movement for individuals or animals who may have been exposed to the virus but are not yet showing symptoms. During an outbreak, individuals who are known to have been in contact with infected animals or people may be placed in quarantine for a period of time to monitor for symptoms. In the case of H5N1, quarantine measures are especially important for those who work in the poultry industry, veterinarians, and individuals who travel to affected areas.

For poultry, quarantine measures may include restricting the movement of birds from infected farms, preventing contact between domestic and wild birds, and imposing travel bans on regions where the virus is widespread. The CDC also works with the U.S. Department of Agriculture (USDA) and state agencies to monitor poultry farms and enforce quarantine measures where necessary.

Testing: Testing is crucial for identifying infected individuals, whether they are human or animal. For humans, the CDC provides diagnostic tools and support to detect H5N1 in clinical settings. This typically involves laboratory tests such as PCR (Polymerase Chain Reaction) to detect the genetic material of the virus, as well as antigen tests to identify the presence of specific proteins.

For animal testing, the CDC works closely with the USDA and other agencies to monitor the health of domestic poultry populations. This includes routine sampling and testing of birds at commercial farms and live bird markets. Early identification of H5N1 in birds allows for rapid intervention, including culling of infected birds to prevent further transmission.

Isolation: Isolation is the practice of separating individuals who are infected with the virus from healthy individuals to prevent the spread of the disease. In a public health context, individuals who are confirmed to be infected with H5N1 are isolated in hospitals or healthcare settings where strict infection control protocols are followed. This is especially important in healthcare settings, where healthcare workers must wear protective equipment such as N95 masks, gloves, and gowns to avoid becoming infected themselves.

During an outbreak, it is also important to isolate infected poultry from healthy birds. This may involve placing sick birds in separate pens or barns, restricting movement, and implementing strict hygiene measures to prevent contamination of surrounding areas.

Isolation efforts are critical to containing the virus and ensuring that it does not spread to other individuals or animals. This is particularly important for H5N1, as it has the potential to spread rapidly and cause severe illness or death in those infected.

Public Health Guidelines for Communities at Risk

Public health guidelines are essential in providing communities with the information and resources they need to protect themselves during an outbreak. For communities at risk of exposure to H5N1, the CDC offers comprehensive guidance on how to minimize the likelihood of infection and respond appropriately if an outbreak occurs.

For individuals living in areas with a high risk of H5N1 infection, the CDC recommends taking several precautionary measures. These include avoiding contact with sick or dead birds, practicing good hygiene (such as frequent handwashing), and avoiding consumption of undercooked poultry products. People who handle birds, particularly in poultry farms or markets, should wear protective equipment to prevent exposure to the virus.

Communities are also encouraged to report any signs of avian influenza in domestic or wild bird populations to local authorities. This early reporting is essential for preventing the spread of the virus and initiating containment measures, such as quarantine and culling.

In the event that a human infection is suspected, individuals should seek medical attention promptly. The CDC emphasizes the importance of rapid diagnostic testing and early treatment with antiviral medications, which can help reduce the severity of the illness and prevent complications.

For healthcare providers, the CDC offers detailed guidelines on how to manage suspected or confirmed cases of H5N1, including isolation protocols, infection control measures, and the use of appropriate personal protective equipment. Healthcare systems in at-risk areas are urged to prepare for potential outbreaks by stockpiling antivirals, ensuring adequate personal protective equipment, and training staff on proper handling of infected individuals.

In addition to these individual measures, the CDC works with local and state governments to ensure that public health systems are prepared to respond to an outbreak. This includes ensuring that public health agencies have the resources and protocols in place to monitor, test, and contain the virus. Public health campaigns are also an essential part of informing the public about the risks of H5N1 and the steps they can take to protect themselves and their families.

Chapter Six: Regional Impacts: The Case of Louisiana and California

A Closer Look at the Louisiana Bird Flu Case

The H5N1 bird flu outbreak that hit Louisiana in 2024 was a significant event that drew national attention due to the severity of the virus and its potential for widespread transmission. Louisiana, with its thriving poultry industry and high concentrations of both domestic and wild birds, became one of the early hot spots for the virus in the United States. The state's poultry farms and commercial bird operations were especially vulnerable to the virus, which thrives in such environments.

The outbreak began in the early months of 2024, when several cases of unusual bird deaths were reported in the rural parts of the state. Initially, these deaths were attributed to natural causes or other avian diseases, but as the number of cases escalated, it became clear that the H5N1 virus was spreading quickly among wild bird populations. In addition to the deaths of domestic poultry, wild birds, including migratory species, were found infected, raising concerns about the virus crossing from animals to humans.

The Louisiana Department of Agriculture and Forestry (LDAF), in collaboration with the CDC and local health departments, immediately launched an investigation. Surveillance teams were deployed to affected areas, and health officials began collecting samples from both domestic and wild bird populations for testing. The state's large agricultural sector meant that millions of poultry birds were potentially at risk, so the response needed to be swift and effective.

As the number of infected farms grew, containment measures were quickly put in place. Quarantine zones were established around farms with confirmed cases, and all affected birds were humanely culled to prevent further spread. These measures aimed not only to limit the virus's transmission but also to prevent the economic damage that would occur from an outbreak of such scale in a state that relies heavily on poultry farming.

In addition to the containment efforts, a public awareness campaign was initiated. Louisiana residents were urged to report any unusual bird deaths, to avoid contact with wild birds, and to follow the guidance of public health officials regarding safety measures. The state also set up emergency response units to handle potential human cases, although no significant human infections were reported in Louisiana during this outbreak. Nevertheless, the situation posed a serious risk, as the virus could have mutated or adapted to human transmission, making it a public health concern for the entire state.

Dr. Daskalakis's Role in the Investigation

Dr. Demetre Daskalakis, as the Director of the Division of Viral Diseases at the CDC, was a key figure in the investigation of the Louisiana bird flu outbreak. His expertise in infectious disease outbreaks and public health management made him an essential part of the response team that coordinated the national effort to track and contain the virus.

Dr. Daskalakis's role involved not just overseeing the CDC's national response to the outbreak but also working directly with state health authorities and local officials in Louisiana. He provided guidance on best practices for surveillance, reporting, and testing, ensuring that all possible cases of infection, whether in humans or animals, were documented and investigated. His leadership was crucial in establishing effective communication channels between the CDC and state health agencies, allowing for a more streamlined and coordinated response.

Additionally, Dr. Daskalakis played a vital role in making expert recommendations about how to handle infected poultry populations. His knowledge of avian influenza allowed him to advise on the necessary measures, including culling, quarantine procedures, and biosecurity protocols for poultry farms. His input ensured that Louisiana's response to the bird flu was consistent with federal guidelines and took into account both human and animal health risks.

Dr. Daskalakis was also a key figure in the public communication strategy. As part of the CDC's efforts to manage public perception and reduce panic, Dr. Daskalakis participated in press briefings and interviews, where he provided expert insight into the situation. He addressed concerns about the potential for human infection, the likelihood of the virus mutating, and the steps being taken to contain the outbreak.

One of Dr. Daskalakis's main priorities was ensuring that the response in Louisiana adhered to scientific evidence and was grounded in public health best practices. By offering his expertise and guidance, he helped the state minimize the risk of a larger outbreak while educating the public about the importance of early detection and reporting. His leadership in Louisiana helped to foster a more effective and organized response to a rapidly evolving public health crisis.

The California State of Emergency: Government Response

California, another state with a high risk of avian influenza transmission due to its large poultry industry and significant migratory bird population, declared a state of emergency in 2024 as the H5N1 virus began to spread. The declaration came after several farms in central and northern California reported cases of bird flu. As in Louisiana, the virus was initially detected in wild birds before moving into commercial poultry operations, raising concerns about both the public health threat and the economic impact of the outbreak.

The state of emergency allowed California's Governor to mobilize additional resources and activate emergency response teams to combat the spread of the virus. The declaration enabled California to access federal funding and resources, including CDC support, to help control the outbreak. This meant that local authorities had more flexibility and authority to implement swift quarantine measures, deploy veterinary teams to inspect poultry farms, and carry out large-scale testing and monitoring programs.

California's public health response was multifaceted. Local authorities immediately imposed restrictions on the movement of birds within affected counties, and farms were ordered to cull infected flocks to prevent the virus from spreading to neighboring farms. Testing centers were set up throughout the state to monitor both wild and domestic bird populations for H5N1. The California Department of Public Health (CDPH) coordinated with the CDC to implement surveillance systems that tracked the spread of the virus among both animal and human populations.

The state's emergency response also involved enhanced public outreach efforts. California health authorities worked with the CDC to educate residents about the risks associated with the bird flu, including how to safely handle birds, report sick animals, and recognize the symptoms of potential human infection. Public service announcements were broadcast on radio and television, urging people to stay informed and take necessary precautions.

Furthermore, California took preventive measures in areas with high concentrations of migratory birds, such as wetlands and bird reserves. The state worked with federal agencies like the U.S. Fish and Wildlife Service to monitor migratory patterns and assess the risk of the virus spreading further. Given California's large agricultural economy, particularly in the poultry industry, the economic impact of an H5N1 outbreak was a major concern. Therefore, efforts to mitigate economic damage were crucial, including compensation for farmers whose flocks had to be culled and financial support to offset losses.

The Role of State Health Authorities in Managing the Outbreak

The role of state health authorities in managing the H5N1 outbreak was central to ensuring that the response was effective and timely. In both Louisiana and California, state health departments played a crucial role in implementing quarantine measures, providing guidance to local authorities, and coordinating with federal agencies like the CDC.

State health authorities were responsible for ensuring that surveillance systems were in place to track the spread of the virus, both in animal and human populations. In Louisiana, for example, the state's Department of Health and Hospitals worked closely with local public health agencies to monitor the situation and offer resources for testing and case management. The state also helped manage the flow of information to the public, ensuring that people were educated on the risks of the virus and the importance of taking precautions.

In California, the Department of Public Health (CDPH) was integral to the state's response. It worked alongside local governments, the CDC, and other health organizations to respond to the outbreak and minimize the risk of human infection. The CDPH's role involved providing expert guidance on public health safety measures, such as the importance of wearing protective gear when handling animals and ensuring that people working with poultry were properly vaccinated.

Both states relied heavily on public-private partnerships to contain the virus. In California, the state government collaborated with the agricultural industry to manage the logistics of bird culling, testing, and surveillance. State health officials also worked with veterinarians, wildlife specialists, and local farmers to ensure that the public health response was as effective as possible.

Ultimately, state health authorities in Louisiana and California played an essential role in containing the H5N1 outbreak by managing quarantine measures, coordinating response efforts, and providing public health guidance. Their work, in collaboration with the CDC and other federal agencies, helped to limit the impact of the virus on public health and agriculture.

Chapter Seven: What We Know and What We Don't: The Unanswered Questions

Understanding the "Spillover" Phenomenon

The "spillover" phenomenon refers to the process by which a disease jumps from one species to another, particularly from animals to humans. In the case of the H5N1 bird flu, the potential for spillover is a major concern. This type of virus is primarily found in birds, particularly wild birds, and can occasionally jump to poultry species. In rare instances, the virus can infect humans, often those in close contact with infected birds, such as poultry workers. The fact that H5N1 can infect multiple species birds, humans, and other mammals—raises the alarm about the potential for future human-to-human transmission, which could lead to a broader pandemic.

Understanding spillover is complex because it depends on a combination of factors, including the characteristics of the virus, the host species, and the environment. In some cases, the virus may mutate in ways that enable it to infect humans more easily, making it far more dangerous. H5N1 is of particular concern due to its high mortality rate in humans, which has led health authorities around the world to monitor and control its spread vigilantly.

Dr. Demetre Daskalakis, in his response to the bird flu outbreak, acknowledged the critical importance of understanding spillover events and their implications for public health. One of the challenges in tracking spillover is the virus's unpredictable nature, while certain strains of avian influenza have the potential to spill over, they may not always do so in a way that leads to human transmission. However, the fact that the virus has spilled over into humans in the past, albeit rarely, indicates that there is a need for constant surveillance, particularly in high-risk areas.

Spillover events are not limited to H5N1. Zoonotic diseases diseases that are transmitted from animals to humans are responsible for some of the deadliest pandemics in history. From HIV/AIDS to the Ebola outbreak, understanding how diseases move between species is crucial in preventing large-scale health crises. Researchers studying spillover focus on the various factors that influence this process, such as animal populations, virus mutations, and human behaviors that increase the likelihood of contact with infected animals.

Dr. Daskalakis emphasized that while human-to-human transmission of H5N1 is rare, the possibility remains a significant public health risk. He called for improved surveillance and research into how viruses like H5N1 spill over into humans and how they can be contained before becoming a major threat.

Why Some Are More at Risk Than Others

One of the key concerns regarding the H5N1 outbreak is why some individuals are more at risk of contracting the virus than others. This disparity is influenced by a combination of biological, environmental, and socioeconomic factors. The virus primarily affects those who come into close contact with infected birds, such as poultry workers, farmers, veterinarians, and people involved in bird trade or farming activities. These individuals are at a higher risk simply because of their proximity to infected animals.

The risk factor also extends to geographical location. Regions with dense poultry farming operations or those near migratory bird routes are more likely to see outbreaks. In the case of Louisiana and California, the high concentration of poultry farming operations and migratory birds made both states particularly vulnerable to the bird flu. People living in these areas or working in the agriculture industry had a significantly higher risk of exposure to the virus.

Another factor contributing to higher risk is the nature of human immune systems. Those with compromised immune systems, such as the elderly, young children, pregnant women, and individuals with pre-existing health conditions, are at a higher risk of severe illness if they contract the virus. In the case of the 2003-2004 H5N1 outbreaks in Southeast Asia, the majority of human cases involved individuals with close exposure to infected birds. However, in some cases, the virus spread to people without direct contact with animals, which raises questions about the virus's potential for broader human-to-human transmission.

Dr. Daskalakis highlighted that while most of the reported cases of H5N1 infection have been limited to those with direct exposure to infected birds, the possibility of new, more virulent strains that could spread more easily among humans remains a serious concern. This is why public health experts continue to emphasize the need for preventive measures and early detection systems to protect those most at risk.

Furthermore, socioeconomic factors play a role in determining who is more likely to be exposed to the virus. Poorer communities, especially in rural areas where poultry farming is a primary source of income, may lack the resources to implement proper biosecurity measures. This lack of access to proper healthcare, hygiene facilities, and education about infection prevention makes these populations more vulnerable to disease outbreaks.

In his statement, Dr. Daskalakis underscored the importance of reaching vulnerable communities and ensuring they have the necessary resources and knowledge to protect themselves from potential outbreaks. This includes promoting hygiene, providing personal protective equipment for workers in high-risk sectors, and improving access to healthcare services.

Research Gaps and the Need for Further Study

Despite the extensive research that has been conducted on avian influenza and other zoonotic diseases, there are still significant gaps in our understanding of how these viruses emerge, spread, and evolve. H5N1, in particular, presents several challenges when it comes to research. For example, the virus's ability to mutate and adapt to new environments means that scientists must constantly monitor changes in the virus's genetic makeup and its potential to cause disease in humans.

One of the key research gaps is understanding how the virus behaves in wild bird populations. Wild birds are natural reservoirs for avian influenza, but because they are difficult to monitor, it is challenging to track the spread of the virus in these populations. Understanding the movement of migratory birds and how they interact with both wild and domestic poultry is crucial for predicting the spread of the virus. Researchers also need to better understand how wild birds can shed the virus in ways that contribute to its transmission to domestic animals and humans.

Another area where research is lacking is in the development of vaccines and antiviral treatments. While there are vaccines available for certain strains of avian influenza, the rapidly evolving nature of the virus means that these vaccines may not always be effective against new variants. Dr. Daskalakis noted the importance of continued research into vaccine development, particularly given the global risks associated with potential pandemics. In addition to vaccines, antiviral medications that can effectively treat human infections caused by H5N1 remain a critical area of study.

Surveillance and early detection systems are also a significant area where research needs to be improved. While the CDC and other global health organizations have made strides in developing monitoring systems for animal and human populations, these systems need to be more robust and interconnected. Early detection of outbreaks in animal populations, followed by rapid response strategies, can prevent the virus from spilling over into human populations.

Dr. Daskalakis emphasized that public health experts must remain vigilant and proactive in addressing research gaps. This includes improving global collaboration on research, ensuring that resources are allocated to high-risk regions, and fostering partnerships between public health agencies, governments, and the private sector.

Dr. Daskalakis's Call for Continued Monitoring and Vigilance

Throughout the 2024 bird flu outbreak, Dr. Daskalakis remained steadfast in his message about the importance of continued vigilance and monitoring. He acknowledged the progress that had been made in controlling the virus but emphasized that the threat of H5N1 and other zoonotic diseases was far from over. He urged both local and global health authorities to remain on high alert for any signs of further mutations or human transmission of the virus.

Dr. Daskalakis also called for increased investment in global health infrastructure, particularly in under-resourced regions that may be more vulnerable to the impacts of outbreaks. He highlighted the importance of preparing for future pandemics by strengthening health systems, investing in research, and improving public health education. His call for continued monitoring and vigilance echoed the lessons learned from previous outbreaks, reminding the global community that public health preparedness is key to managing and preventing future health crises.

In his statement, Dr. Daskalakis stressed the need for comprehensive surveillance systems that monitor both animal and human health. This includes the use of advanced technology to track the spread of viruses in real-time and the development of predictive models that can help anticipate future outbreaks. He also emphasized the importance of sharing data across borders, as pandemics are global threats that require a coordinated response.

By maintaining a focus on research, preparedness, and international cooperation, Dr. Daskalakis believes that the global community can reduce the risk of future pandemics and better manage outbreaks when they do occur.

Chapter Eight: Risk to the Public: Analyzing Dr. Daskalakis's Risk Assessment

How the CDC Determines Risk Levels

The Centers for Disease Control and Prevention (CDC) plays a pivotal role in determining the risk levels of emerging diseases such as the H5N1 bird flu. Through a comprehensive risk assessment process, the CDC evaluates numerous factors to gauge the severity of an outbreak and the potential threat it poses to the public. This assessment not only includes the biological characteristics of the virus itself but also takes into account external variables such as human behavior, environmental conditions, and existing public health infrastructure. The goal is to understand the full scope of the threat and create appropriate response strategies.

The process begins with monitoring and surveillance. The CDC relies on global reporting systems to track outbreaks, including data from both human and animal populations. In the case of H5N1, this includes tracking the virus's presence in wild and domestic bird populations, as well as identifying any human infections. By monitoring patterns of infection, scientists are able to detect unusual spikes in cases or the emergence of new strains that may pose a greater risk.

Once an outbreak is identified, the CDC considers several core factors when determining the risk level:

1. Transmission Potential: One of the first and most important factors in risk assessment is how the virus spreads. The CDC evaluates whether the virus is primarily spread through animal-to-human transmission or if it can spread more easily between humans. The risk of a pandemic increases significantly if the virus can mutate to enable human-to-human transmission. For H5N1, the virus has primarily been transmitted from birds to humans, but the possibility of mutations that allow human-to-human transmission is always a concern.

2. Severity of Disease: The severity of the disease is also a critical factor. H5N1 is highly pathogenic in birds, and while it does not always cause severe illness in humans, when it does, it can lead to high mortality rates. The CDC monitors the fatality rates in human cases to assess how dangerous the virus is in the population.

3. Geographic Spread: The CDC assesses the spread of the virus geographically, considering factors such as migration patterns of wild birds and the movement of poultry, which can influence how widely the virus can spread. If the outbreak is localized to specific regions with few global connections, the risk is contained; however, if it spreads to major urban areas or through international trade routes, the threat increases.

4. Public Health Capacity: An outbreak's risk is also determined by the capacity of the affected region's healthcare system to respond. This includes the availability of medical supplies, the readiness of public health infrastructure, and the ability to conduct mass vaccinations or distribute antiviral treatments if necessary. Regions with well-prepared health systems can handle an outbreak more effectively, reducing the risk to the public.

Dr. Demetre Daskalakis, as a senior figure within the CDC, emphasized that rapid and efficient response is key to minimizing the risk associated with infectious diseases like H5N1. The CDC's risk assessment process is critical in guiding public health decisions, including the deployment of vaccines, the imposition of quarantine measures, and the provision of public health recommendations.

The Role of Age, Health Conditions, and Exposure

When assessing risk during an outbreak like the H5N1 bird flu, one of the primary factors the CDC considers is the population's susceptibility to infection. This includes how age, health conditions, and levels of exposure to the virus influence an individual's likelihood of contracting the disease, as well as the severity of the illness if they do become infected.

1. Age: Certain age groups are more vulnerable to infectious diseases. The very young, the elderly, and pregnant women often have weaker immune systems, making them more susceptible to severe illness or death if they contract a virus like H5N1. In particular, young children may have developing immune systems that are less capable of fighting off infection, while older adults may have compromised immune systems due to age-related factors or pre-existing health conditions.

2. Health Conditions: Individuals with chronic health conditions such as asthma, diabetes, heart disease, or autoimmune disorders are more vulnerable during an outbreak. These pre-existing conditions can impair the body's ability to fight off infections, making individuals with compromised health systems more likely to experience severe symptoms or complications. In the

case of H5N1, a viral respiratory infection, individuals with respiratory conditions or weakened lung function are particularly at risk.

3. Exposure: The most significant factor in determining the risk of contracting H5N1 is exposure to infected animals, particularly birds. People who work in close proximity to poultry, such as farmers, veterinarians, and workers in live bird markets, are at a much higher risk than the general population. Even for individuals who do not work directly with animals, those living in or near affected areas or traveling to regions with known outbreaks may face increased exposure risks. Dr. Daskalakis's statement reflected the importance of public health recommendations to avoid contact with sick birds and to ensure that poultry products are properly cooked.

Understanding the interplay between these factors allows public health officials to prioritize resources and determine who is most at risk during an outbreak. Dr. Daskalakis noted that during an outbreak, measures should be taken to protect the most vulnerable populations, ensuring they have access to preventive treatments such as vaccines or antiviral medications, and that they receive proper education on how to reduce their exposure to the virus.

Public Behavior and Precautionary Measures

Public behavior plays a significant role in the spread of infectious diseases. During a bird flu outbreak, how people respond to public health advisories and how they alter their daily behavior can have a direct impact on how the virus spreads. In his statement, Dr. Daskalakis highlighted the importance of precautionary measures in reducing transmission rates and ensuring that the virus does not evolve into a pandemic.

One of the most effective measures in controlling the spread of H5N1 is avoiding contact with infected birds. The CDC and other health agencies issue warnings to limit exposure to poultry farms, live bird markets, and other high-risk areas where the virus is most likely to be found. Dr. Daskalakis emphasized the importance of public health education, urging people to follow safety guidelines and report any sick or dead birds to local authorities. He noted that while the risk of human-to-human transmission of H5N1 is low, human behaviors such as improper handling of poultry or consumption of undercooked bird products can increase the risk of infection.

In addition to limiting exposure, personal hygiene is another important factor in reducing the spread of the virus. Public health recommendations include regular handwashing, wearing personal protective equipment for those in high-risk occupations, and ensuring that proper sanitation measures are followed in areas where the virus is prevalent. Public health agencies also advocate for strict biosecurity measures in poultry farming and the culling of infected animals to prevent further spread of the virus.

While individual behaviors are critical in controlling the spread, community-wide measures, such as quarantine and isolation, also play an essential role in limiting exposure. Dr. Daskalakis emphasized that widespread public compliance with health recommendations and a coordinated response from local, state, and federal health authorities are necessary to reduce the risks posed by an outbreak.

The Reality of Person-to-Person Transmission

One of the most concerning aspects of any emerging infectious disease is the potential for person-to-person transmission. While the primary mode of transmission for H5N1 has been animal-to-human, there have been isolated cases in which the virus has spread from one human to another. This is extremely rare and is typically associated with close, prolonged contact between individuals, such as in a household where an infected person is caring for a sick family member.

The CDC monitors any instances of person-to-person transmission to determine whether the virus has mutated in a way that allows it to spread more easily between humans. If H5N1 were to mutate and become capable of sustained human-to-human transmission, it could lead to a far more widespread outbreak with a much greater impact on public health. Dr. Daskalakis cautioned that while the risk of widespread person-to-person transmission of H5N1 remains low, it is a constant concern for public health officials, and this risk must be actively monitored.

Dr. Daskalakis emphasized the need for continued vigilance and preparedness in the event that person-to-person transmission of H5N1 becomes more common. He underscored the importance of global surveillance systems, which track mutations in the virus and monitor any signs of increased transmission capabilities. The ability to detect changes in the virus's behavior at an early stage is essential in preventing larger outbreaks and protecting public health.

Chapter Nine: Preparing for the Future: Lessons from the H5N1 Outbreak

Global Health Security and Pandemic Preparedness

The H5N1 bird flu outbreak serves as a reminder of the ongoing challenges in global health security and the importance of pandemic preparedness. Infectious diseases such as H5N1 can spread rapidly across borders, creating health, social, and economic crises. Global health security is not only about responding to current outbreaks, but also about ensuring that the global community is prepared for the threats that may arise in the future. This requires international collaboration, investment in health infrastructure, and a commitment to surveillance and early warning systems that can detect outbreaks before they escalate.

One of the key components of global health security is the ability to share information and coordinate responses. During the 2024 H5N1 outbreak, the World Health Organization (WHO), national health authorities like the CDC, and other organizations worked together to track the virus, share data, and implement containment strategies. However, the rapid spread of diseases like H5N1 highlights the gaps that still exist in communication and coordination between countries. Effective global health security requires timely information exchange and the capacity to respond quickly at the international level.

Pandemic preparedness involves not only robust surveillance systems but also an adequate response infrastructure. Governments must have systems in place to ensure that health care workers are trained, supplies are available, and emergency response plans are ready to be activated. This includes building stockpiles of antiviral medications, vaccines, and personal protective equipment, as well as ensuring that there are established protocols for quarantine and isolation if necessary. These preparations should also involve investing in infrastructure that can handle the surge in medical cases that often accompanies an outbreak.

The COVID-19 pandemic demonstrated the severe consequences of underestimating the global threat of infectious diseases. In contrast, the 2024 H5N1 outbreak has underscored the importance of learning from past mistakes and taking proactive steps toward pandemic preparedness. Dr. Demetre Daskalakis, in his official statement, emphasized the need for ongoing investments in pandemic preparedness, urging governments to consider future risks, not just immediate threats. This approach involves enhancing surveillance networks, strengthening public health systems, and fostering international partnerships to ensure a coordinated global response.

As Dr. Daskalakis has pointed out, "the best way to prepare for a pandemic is to invest in preparedness, not just response." This foresight is crucial to improving global health security and minimizing the impact of future outbreaks.

The CDC's Long-Term Vision for Handling Avian Influenza

The CDC has a crucial role in managing outbreaks of avian influenza, and its long-term vision includes not only responding to current outbreaks like H5N1 but also working toward preventing future ones. In the wake of the 2024 outbreak, the CDC's strategy focuses on three main areas: surveillance, containment, and prevention.

Surveillance is the backbone of the CDC's approach. The CDC's system for monitoring avian influenza is designed to detect the virus in both animals and humans, identifying potential risks before they escalate into a full-blown outbreak. The CDC collaborates with other national and international organizations, such as the World Organization for Animal Health (OIE) and the WHO, to track the spread of the virus across different regions. By using cutting-edge technology and data analysis, the CDC aims to identify areas of concern and implement preventative measures quickly.

Containment involves responding rapidly when the virus is detected in animals or humans. The CDC has developed a series of protocols for containment, including culling infected poultry, implementing quarantines, and issuing travel advisories if necessary. During the 2024 H5N1 outbreak, the CDC worked closely with local authorities to implement these measures, limiting the virus's spread and preventing it from becoming a larger crisis. These measures are part of a broader strategy to reduce the impact of future outbreaks and ensure that health systems are not overwhelmed.

Prevention, however, is the long-term goal of the CDC's strategy. The CDC is working on developing vaccines and antiviral treatments that can prevent or reduce the severity of infection in both humans and animals. Efforts are also being made to enhance biosecurity measures in poultry farming, ensuring that H5N1 and other avian influenza viruses are contained within animal populations. These prevention efforts are critical in the ongoing battle against avian influenza, especially as the virus continues to evolve and potentially poses a greater risk to public health.

Another critical aspect of the CDC's long-term vision is education and communication. Dr. Daskalakis emphasized the need for clear, accurate communication to the public and healthcare providers regarding the risks of avian influenza. By providing consistent updates, sharing data on the virus's spread, and educating communities about preventive measures, the CDC aims to empower individuals and communities to take appropriate action.

Dr. Daskalakis's work with the CDC in response to H5N1 exemplifies the agency's commitment to addressing the immediate threat while preparing for future challenges. His vision for handling avian influenza reflects a holistic approach that includes not just surveillance and containment, but also long-term research and global collaboration to mitigate the risk of future pandemics.

Lessons Learned from the 2024 Outbreak and Future Risks

The 2024 H5N1 outbreak provided valuable lessons about the challenges and complexities of managing an infectious disease outbreak. One of the most important lessons learned was the importance of early detection and rapid response. The sooner an outbreak is identified, the more effectively it can be contained, preventing widespread transmission and minimizing its impact. However, the outbreak also highlighted some of the limitations in global surveillance systems, underscoring the need for improvements in data sharing and real-time monitoring.

The outbreak also highlighted the role of communication in preventing panic and confusion. Dr. Daskalakis emphasized that transparent and clear communication is essential during any health crisis. By keeping the public informed and providing actionable advice, health authorities can reduce anxiety and help people make informed decisions about how to protect themselves and their families. One of the challenges faced during the 2024 outbreak was managing public perception and combating misinformation about the virus, which in some cases led to unnecessary panic. Lessons from this will be essential in improving the communication strategies during future outbreaks.

Another critical lesson from the 2024 outbreak was the need for more robust global collaboration. While national responses were coordinated, the global nature of infectious diseases demands stronger partnerships across borders. The H5N1 outbreak has reinforced the importance of sharing information, resources, and expertise in combating global health threats. In particular, the involvement of international agencies, such as the WHO and the OIE, is crucial in managing future risks and ensuring that countries can respond effectively.

Future risks associated with H5N1 and other avian influenza strains remain significant. The virus continues to evolve, and while human-to-human transmission is still limited, the possibility exists for a more transmissible strain to emerge. As such, it is essential to continue monitoring the virus, investing in research, and preparing for the worst-case scenario. Dr. Daskalakis's statement underscored the need for vigilance, even as the immediate threat of the 2024 outbreak wanes.

How Communities Can Prepare for Future Outbreaks

While governments and public health agencies play a significant role in managing outbreaks, communities also have an essential part to play in preparedness efforts. Dr. Daskalakis stressed that local communities need to be proactive in their approach to pandemic preparedness. By understanding the risks and taking preventive measures, individuals can help reduce the spread of disease and support broader public health efforts.

First and foremost, communities should focus on education and awareness. Public health agencies like the CDC can provide resources to educate individuals about the risks of avian influenza and the steps they can take to protect themselves. This includes basic hygiene practices, such as washing hands frequently and avoiding contact with sick animals, as well as more specific recommendations for people who live in or near poultry farms.

Second, communities should work to strengthen their local health systems. This includes ensuring that healthcare providers are equipped with the necessary training and resources to respond to outbreaks effectively. It also means building partnerships with local governments, public health agencies, and community organizations to ensure that there is a coordinated response to any potential outbreak.

Finally, communities can prepare by developing and practicing response plans. This might include setting up community emergency response teams, establishing communication channels for disseminating information, and organizing local volunteers to assist in response efforts. Dr. Daskalakis emphasized that community-level preparedness can make a significant difference in the speed and effectiveness of a response.

Chapter Ten: Beyond the Bird Flu: Dr. Daskalakis's Broader Impact on Public Health

Dr. Daskalakis's Contributions to Infectious Disease Control

Dr. Demetre Daskalakis's contributions to the field of infectious disease control are vast and have had a significant impact on public health not only in the United States but also on a global scale. His career, which spans various critical roles in public health, has been focused on preventing, controlling, and managing infectious diseases, with an emphasis on understanding the factors that drive their spread and the strategies that can be employed to mitigate them.

One of Dr. Daskalakis's earliest contributions was in the realm of HIV/AIDS prevention and management. During his time at the Centers for Disease Control and Prevention (CDC), he played an instrumental role in designing public health programs aimed at reducing the spread of HIV. His work included improving testing, counseling, and prevention strategies, as well as addressing the social and structural factors that contribute to higher rates of transmission, such as stigma and lack of access to healthcare. This experience helped Dr. Daskalakis understand the intricate interplay between societal factors and disease transmission, which would prove invaluable when addressing other infectious diseases like the bird flu.

As the Deputy Director for the CDC's Division of Viral Diseases, Dr. Daskalakis became a central figure in the United States' response to emerging infectious diseases, including viral outbreaks like Zika, Ebola, and COVID-19. His expertise in communicable diseases and public health response was critical in shaping the nation's approach to these global health crises. He advocated for stronger surveillance systems, greater investment in vaccines, and more robust community-level interventions. His leadership in this capacity ensured that the CDC could respond effectively and efficiently when threats like Zika and Ebola emerged.

During the 2024 H5N1 bird flu outbreak, Dr. Daskalakis once again demonstrated his invaluable leadership in infectious disease control. As the CDC's point person on this outbreak, he played a critical role in assessing the risk, providing guidance to local health departments, and helping to shape the national response. His expertise in surveillance and containment strategies helped to minimize the spread of the virus. Additionally, his insights into the dynamics of zoonotic diseases, diseases that can spread from animals to humans, allowed health officials to better understand how H5N1 could potentially escalate and what measures would be most effective in curbing its transmission.

Beyond specific outbreaks, Dr. Daskalakis's work in infectious disease control has left a lasting imprint on the public health field. His advocacy for research into new diagnostic tools and vaccines, as well as his calls for greater international cooperation in disease monitoring, have pushed the boundaries of what is possible in controlling infectious diseases. His contributions to developing frameworks for global health preparedness and response have laid the groundwork for a more resilient public health system capable of facing future pandemics.

Advancing Public Health Policy

Dr. Daskalakis's impact on public health extends beyond his work in disease control; he has also played a pivotal role in advancing public health policy. Throughout his career, Dr. Daskalakis has been a tireless advocate for policies that address the root causes of health disparities and promote equitable access to healthcare for all individuals. His belief in the power of policy to shape health outcomes has driven many of his professional endeavors, particularly in relation to infectious diseases and the public health system's capacity to respond to outbreaks.

In his leadership role at the CDC, Dr. Daskalakis worked to influence health policy at both the national and local levels. One of his key contributions was his emphasis on integrating public health responses into broader governmental and societal structures. He advocated for policies that not only address immediate health concerns but also focus on building long-term public health infrastructure that can withstand future crises. For example, during the COVID-19 pandemic, he played a significant role in promoting the need for coordinated policies that ensure a rapid and effective response to health emergencies, such as universal access to vaccines, fair distribution of medical resources, and improved healthcare workforce preparedness.

Dr. Daskalakis also pushed for more inclusive public health policies that take into account the social determinants of health factors like income inequality, housing instability, and access to education, which disproportionately affect marginalized communities. In the case of H5N1 and other zoonotic diseases, his policy work often intersected with environmental health, as he called for stronger regulations on animal farming practices, better monitoring of potential reservoirs for disease, and policies that reduce the risk of outbreaks in vulnerable regions.

Perhaps one of Dr. Daskalakis's most significant policy contributions was his advocacy for the prioritization of infectious disease research and preparedness funding. He understood that in a rapidly globalizing world, new and emerging diseases pose an ongoing threat to public health. As such, he has been a leading voice in calling for consistent funding and long-term investments in research and public health infrastructure, rather than just responding reactively to outbreaks. His policy work has been instrumental in shaping the way the United States approaches global health challenges and positioning public health agencies to be more proactive and less reactive.

In addition to his work on infectious diseases, Dr. Daskalakis has been a strong advocate for mental health services as part of broader public health policy. In many outbreaks, such as the Zika and Ebola crises, mental health has often been overlooked despite the emotional and psychological toll these events take on individuals and communities. Dr. Daskalakis has consistently emphasized the need for integrated approaches to public health that prioritize both physical and mental well-being, helping shape policies that support mental health resources during and after public health emergencies.

The Role of Leadership in Managing Health Crises

Dr. Daskalakis's leadership during times of crisis highlights the crucial role that strong, informed, and compassionate leadership plays in managing public health emergencies. His ability to manage complex situations, make critical decisions under pressure, and communicate effectively with both the public and other health officials has earned him respect in the field of public health.

Effective leadership in public health is not just about managing the technical aspects of an outbreak, such as data collection, surveillance, and containment measures; it also involves guiding people through uncertainty, addressing public concerns, and maintaining trust in health institutions. Dr. Daskalakis's leadership style emphasizes transparency, collaboration, and preparation. During the 2024 H5N1 outbreak, he communicated clearly with the public and the media, offering insights into the status of the outbreak and the steps being taken to mitigate the spread of the virus. His willingness to engage with the media and the public helped demystify complex health concepts and reduced the fear and anxiety that often accompanies such crises.

In addition to his communication skills, Dr. Daskalakis has demonstrated the importance of collaboration in leadership. Public health crises do not occur in a vacuum, and Dr. Daskalakis recognizes the importance of working across sectors to ensure an effective response. This includes collaborating with local and state health departments, international health agencies, and non-governmental organizations to ensure that response efforts are coordinated, resources are allocated effectively, and policies are aligned. Dr. Daskalakis's leadership in these areas has proven to be invaluable in the fight against infectious diseases, ensuring that the response is both comprehensive and equitable.

Another key aspect of Dr. Daskalakis's leadership is his focus on preparation. Leadership in public health is not just about reacting to crises but also about preventing them. His work in shaping the CDC's long-term vision for pandemic preparedness is a testament to his commitment to future-proofing public health systems. He has consistently advocated for policies that emphasize the importance of training, resource allocation, and system design that can withstand future health challenges. His leadership has helped position public health agencies to respond not only to known threats but also to anticipate and mitigate emerging risks.

Finally, Dr. Daskalakis's leadership extends beyond technical expertise. His commitment to equity and the inclusion of diverse perspectives in public health decision-making is a cornerstone of his approach. He has often highlighted the need to ensure that marginalized communities, including racial and ethnic minorities, LGBTQ+ individuals, and those in low-income settings, are not left behind during outbreaks and are provided with the resources and support they need to stay safe. His leadership has helped shape a more inclusive approach to public health that values every individual's health and well-being.

In conclusion, Dr. Demetre Daskalakis's contributions to public health are far-reaching, encompassing infectious disease control, public health policy advancement, and crisis leadership. His work has not only shaped the response to specific health crises but has also influenced the broader field of public health, laying the foundation for a more resilient, equitable, and proactive approach to health emergencies. Through his leadership, Dr. Daskalakis has demonstrated that effective public health management requires a comprehensive approach that integrates research, policy, community engagement, and global collaboration. His broader impact on public health will continue to influence future generations of health professionals, researchers, and policymakers as they work to address the ever-evolving challenges of global health.

Conclusion

Throughout his distinguished career, Dr. Demetre Daskalakis has made significant contributions to the field of public health, particularly in the area of infectious disease control. His work has been instrumental in shaping the United States' response to some of the most critical health crises of our time, including HIV/AIDS, the Zika virus, and the ongoing fight against pandemics like COVID-19 and the 2024 H5N1 bird flu outbreak. Dr. Daskalakis's deep understanding of infectious diseases, coupled with his strong leadership abilities, has made him a key figure in shaping both national and global responses to public health emergencies.

One of his major contributions lies in the integration of epidemiology, public health policy, and effective communication. As Deputy Director of the CDC's Division of Viral Diseases, Dr. Daskalakis has consistently advocated for the development of better surveillance systems and the use of data-driven strategies to monitor and control the spread of infectious diseases. His leadership was critical in organizing and executing effective containment measures during viral outbreaks, ensuring that resources were efficiently allocated, and guiding the public on necessary health precautions.

Dr. Daskalakis's work on the 2024 H5N1 bird flu outbreak exemplifies his unique approach to infectious disease response. His timely statement on the risk assessment of H5N1, the evaluation of its transmission potential, and the public's health guidance provided clarity and reassurance during a period of uncertainty. Through his insights, Dr. Daskalakis underscored the importance of early detection, quarantine measures, and the development of vaccines, which were essential to preventing the wider spread of the virus.

Moreover, his continued emphasis on the interconnectedness of human health, animal health, and the environment has been fundamental in advancing public health practices. This holistic approach, which he applied to both the HIV/AIDS epidemic and the bird flu crisis, encourages governments and public health agencies to take a comprehensive stance when addressing infectious diseases. His recognition of the broader social, economic, and environmental factors that influence health has resulted in public health strategies that prioritize the inclusion of all sectors, from agriculture to social services.

Dr. Daskalakis's ability to foster collaboration among various health organizations and his commitment to transparency during times of crisis have further cemented his role as a leader in global health. His efforts to mobilize resources during health emergencies, provide guidance to local health authorities, and offer reassurance to the public have left an indelible mark on the health landscape.

The Role of Expert Voices in Shaping Public Health Responses

In the modern world, the role of expert voices in shaping public health responses cannot be overstated. Dr. Daskalakis's contributions to public health exemplify why expert opinions are essential in managing infectious diseases and shaping global health strategies. During health crises such as the H5N1 outbreak and the COVID-19 pandemic, it is the expertise of individuals like Dr. Daskalakis that ensures accurate information is disseminated to the public, helping to guide behavior, influence policy decisions, and promote public trust in health institutions.

Expert voices provide not only the technical knowledge necessary to understand and combat emerging health threats but also the leadership and communication skills needed to navigate the complexities of a crisis. Public health experts like Dr. Daskalakis help clarify the science behind infectious diseases and recommend strategies to contain them. They also play a crucial role in reassuring the public and preventing panic by offering well-reasoned, scientifically backed responses to health emergencies. Their guidance ensures that government agencies, international organizations, and the public remain focused on the most critical actions required to safeguard health.

In addition to their technical expertise, public health experts also influence policy at the highest levels. Dr. Daskalakis's work has demonstrated how expert voices can drive policy changes that improve the public health infrastructure, ensure timely interventions, and foster collaboration across borders. For example, his work with the CDC has directly influenced the formulation of national policies regarding vaccination programs, disease surveillance, and global health security measures. His advocacy for policies that integrate social determinants of health, mental health considerations, and healthcare access further illustrates how experts can shape policy to be more inclusive and responsive to the needs of diverse populations.

The credibility and reliability of experts are particularly important in the age of misinformation, where misleading claims and conspiracy theories can undermine public health efforts. In this context, trusted voices like Dr. Daskalakis become a cornerstone of effective crisis communication. Their ability to engage with both the media and the public in clear and understandable terms fosters a sense of trust and empowers individuals to make informed decisions about their health. Without the guidance of experts, public health responses may lack coordination, transparency, and effectiveness.

In light of these factors, Dr. Daskalakis's leadership serves as a reminder of the immense value that expert opinions bring to the table. Whether in the development of surveillance tools, the design of public health policies, or the implementation of preventive measures, experts play a central role in shaping responses to health threats and ensuring the safety and well-being of communities.

Final Thoughts on the Global Health Landscape

The global health landscape is one that is increasingly interconnected and complex, with emerging infectious diseases continuing to pose a significant threat to public health worldwide. From zoonotic diseases like H5N1 and COVID-19 to antibiotic resistance and the ongoing challenge of controlling chronic diseases, the future of global health requires a concerted effort from governments, international organizations, healthcare providers, and the public.

As the world continues to battle existing health challenges and prepare for potential new threats, the role of public health leaders like Dr. Daskalakis will be essential in guiding responses and shaping policies. His work, particularly in the context of the H5N1 outbreak, has underscored the importance of global collaboration, early detection systems, and the need for strong health infrastructures capable of responding swiftly to emerging threats. Dr. Daskalakis's vision for a comprehensive approach to public health, one that integrates disease prevention, health equity, and sustainable health systems remains a critical component of future efforts to combat pandemics and other health crises.

In addition, the experience of past outbreaks, including those under Dr. Daskalakis's leadership, has highlighted the importance of preparedness. While global health organizations like the World Health Organization (WHO) and the CDC have made great strides in improving pandemic preparedness, much work remains to be done to strengthen global health security. National governments must continue to prioritize funding for research, invest in public health infrastructure, and promote international cooperation in disease surveillance and response.

The COVID-19 pandemic and the H5N1 outbreak have made it clear that global health security is not just a national concern but a shared responsibility. Disease outbreaks do not respect borders, and the ability of one country to effectively manage an outbreak can significantly impact global health. As such, it is imperative that nations collaborate more effectively in building global health frameworks that can respond swiftly to health threats and reduce the burden of disease worldwide.

Finally, the future of global health will require ongoing vigilance and the ability to adapt to changing circumstances. New technologies, improved diagnostic tools, and more efficient vaccine development are all promising advancements that will enhance our ability to respond to health crises. However, without the leadership, expertise, and commitment of individuals like Dr. Daskalakis, these advancements alone will not be enough to protect global populations from the next wave of infectious diseases. The key to success will be in leveraging expert voices, fostering international collaboration, and continuously learning from past experiences to build a healthier, more resilient world.

In conclusion, Dr. Daskalakis's contributions to public health, particularly in infectious disease control, provide a valuable blueprint for managing the global health challenges of the future. His insights into the complexities of disease transmission, risk assessment, and the role of expert voices in shaping public health responses will continue to guide future efforts to protect public health. The ongoing fight against emerging health threats is one that requires dedication, collaboration, and a long-term commitment to building robust and adaptable health systems. As we look to the future, Dr. Daskalakis's work reminds us that public health is a shared responsibility and that, together, we can address the health challenges of tomorrow.

www.ingramcontent.com/pod-product-compliance
Lightning Source LLC
Chambersburg PA
CBHW050323230526
45471CB00005B/2326